Starting Points

The Basics of Understanding and Supporting Children and Youth with Asperger Syndrome

Jill Hudson

Brenda Smith Myles

APC

Autism Asperger Publishing Co.
P.O. Box 23173
Shawnee Mission, Kansas 66283-0173
www.asperger.net

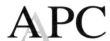

© 2007 Autism Asperger Publishing Co.
P.O. Box 23173
Shawnee Mission, Kansas 66283-0173
www.asperger.net • 913.897.1004

Publisher's Cataloging-in-Publication

Hudson, Jill.

    Starting points : the basics of understanding and supporting children and youth with Asperger syndrome/ Jill Hudson, Brenda Smith Myles. -- 1st ed. -- Shawnee Mission, Kan. : Autism Asperger Pub. Co., c2007.

        p. ; cm.

        ISBN: 978-1-934575-08-6
        LCCN: 2007933729
        Includes bibliographical references.

        1. Asperger's syndrome in children. 2. Asperger's syndrome in adolescence. 3. Asperger's syndrome in children--Treatment. 4. Asperger's syndrome in adolescence--Treatment. I. Myles, Brenda Smith. I. Title. II. How to understand and support children and youth with Asperger Syndrome.

RJ506.A9 H83 2007
618.92/858832--dc22   0709

This book is designed in Frutiger and Jimbo.

Printed in the United States of America.

Cover background art: ©iStockphoto.com/Alejandro Raymond

Table of Contents

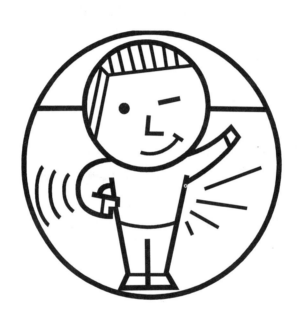

Introduction

Since you have picked up this book, we assume that you have just begun the adventuresome journey of living or working with an individual with Asperger Syndrome (AS). You may be a parent, teacher, relative, community member, or friend. The individual may be a 4-year-old child or an 11-year-old on the brink of adolescence. Regardless of your specific role or the age of the child with AS, you care enough to learn more about his or her unique characteristics and needs in hopes of being able to provide help and support.

This book is intended to assist you in this important endeavor. Each section of the book presents an introductory overview of a major characteristic of AS. No two individuals with AS are the same, so it is important to keep in mind that these characteristics may appear differently in each person. We have tried to provide you with a global perspective on how the various characteristics may overlap with one another and how they may manifest themselves in a variety of situations.

The following table highlights actions or preferences that you may see demonstrated by the individual with AS. They are grouped according to the category in which they are further discussed in the text. Paired with the explanation of each characteristic, you will find several bulleted interventions. These are suggestions that we hope you will implement at home, at school, and in the community.

Actions or Preferences That You May See in an Individual with Asperger Syndrome

Seeing the Big Picture
Child may ...
- Have difficulty taking the perspective of others
- Have difficulty with abstract concepts and thoughts

Self-Regulation
Child may ...
- Have a preferred item or routine that provides comfort
- Be sensitive to even the tiniest stimuli in the environment
- Have difficulty regulating sensory-rich environments
- Have difficulty organizing information and routines
- Show raised levels of anxiety
- Have difficulty understanding and regulating emotions
- Easily escalate into a meltdown if he cannot regulate emotions or reaction to a situation

Structure and Predictability
Child may ...
- Prefer structure and sameness
- Need explanations for transitions or changes in schedule
- Like to anticipate and predict the steps in the routine
- Prefer advanced notice or warning about individual steps in a process, change in routine, or an upcoming transition

Understanding the Thoughts and Feelings of Others
Child may ...
- Fail to directly answer questions
- Be unable to understand the inferred meaning of idioms, metaphors, or comparisons
- Not understand sarcasm or jokes
- Be a literal thinker or interpreter of words
- Have difficulty recognizing and interpreting facial cues, body language, voice inflection, and gestures
- Have difficulty recognizing, interpreting, and empathizing with the emotions of others

Getting Along with Others: Social Interactions
Child may ...
- Talk about unusual subjects
- Refer to a script to converse or answer questions
- Find it easier to answer questions with choices versus open-ended questions

Unwritten Rules

Child may ...
- Be unaware of the subtle customs within a given environment
- Fail to realize that choices are available if not specifically stated
- Appear oblivious to common sense routines and occurrences

Special or Unique Interests

Child may ...
- Have a strong preferred special interest
- Converse with self or imaginary figures

Organization

Child may ...
- Have difficulty organizing information and routines

Daily Living Skills

Child may ...
- Have difficulty retaining and following verbal instructions
- Need cues for how and when to transition from an activity or place to the next

School Subjects

Child may ...
- Prefer visual directions or instructions instead of verbal ones
- Find it easier to answer questions with choices versus open-ended questions
- Need to be asked one question at a time, eliciting a concrete answer
- May vary in level across domains, excelling in one area and showing deficits in another

Note. There is overlap between some of the categories.

Adapted from Hudson, J. (2006). *Prescriptions for success: Supporting children with autism spectrum disorders in the medical environment* (p. 22). Shawnee Mission, KS: Autism Asperger Publishing Company. Used with permission.

Not all interventions will work the first time, nor with every child, so be persistent in looking for what works best for you and the individual. Some interventions are very simple and others require a little more thought and planning to carry out, but there is sure to be something applicable to your setting and the child you are working or living with. The suggestions are research-based and have been shown to support individuals with AS over and over again.

We hope that you will find this book a useful resource, frequently visited and easily implemented. By creating consistency across settings and sharing successful ideas with others who engage and interact with the child or youth, you are building a foundation for success and a community that will continue to enrich the child and be enriched, in turn.

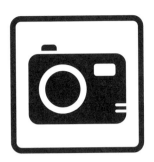

Seeing the Big Picture

Many individuals with AS react and interact with the world from a single point of view – their own. They focus on details and often miss how they themselves are intertwined with and impact the greater world around them.

It is difficult to have a perspective of others if you are not aware of your own actions and thoughts, as illustrated in the following example.

When asked what he was thinking about while walking down the hallway out of line, Lewis replied, "I don't know." In reality, Lewis probably does not remember what he was daydreaming about or why he was not walking in line with his classmates. Even when repeatedly asked why he was out of line, Lewis still does not remember. This is because he was not aware of being out of line or daydreaming while walking down the hall.

No amount of persistence will enable him to recall the scene. Lewis is not being obstinate or defiant. He was not self-aware and, therefore, was unable to monitor his actions and thoughts. If he cannot monitor his actions and thoughts, he cannot regulate them. And if he cannot regulate them, he cannot determine how they affect others around him. Each of these skills must be taught and mastered individually.

Perspective taking includes not only an awareness of one's own thoughts, percep-tions, and ideas, but also an awareness of the potential thoughts, perceptions, and ideas of those around. Such awareness allows one to recognize and predict how one's actions and reactions influence a situation or other people. It also allows one to step into the shoes of another person and see the world through his or her eyes.

Strategies for Helping to See the Big Picture

✔ **Direct Teaching** – Assist the child in determining what occurs in the world around him. Point out what others are doing and show how their actions af-fect his reaction. Help him to be aware of what he is doing, how he is acting, and how he influences others around him.

Give him a role or responsibility on which to focus and "self-monitor" during a short task, such as holding two ice cream cones while the parent pays for the ice cream and then takes one of the cones back from the child. The child's role is to carefully hold two cones and not move. When he has accomplished this task, he has become aware of his behavior and the control he has over himself.

As the child becomes more aware of his behaviors, his responsibility to regu-late those behaviors may be increased. That is, as he is more aware of his ac-tions, he is expected to be more accountable for regulating those actions. As his ability to regulate becomes more consistent, paralleling his level of aware-ness, his ability to assess a situation and behave/react accordingly increases, too. Such assessment eventually leads the child to a greater understanding of the world around him and the multiple perspectives of others.

✔ **Video Modeling** – Use a video camera to capture an interaction between a child and some friends or family members. Review the footage with the child and narrate the interactions, one by one, as they happen. Ask the child ques-tions about his own behaviors as well as the behaviors of the others in the scene. Listen to the perspective that he provides. Continue pointing out cues and clues that provide insight and more perspective on the situation. For example, "When you did not go over to Kimmie and Miguel and ask if you could join their game of *Chutes and Ladders*, they continued to play by themselves because they did not know that you wanted to play with them. What can you do next time you want to play?"

☑ **SOCCSS** – Use this problem-solving strategy (see page 8) to review the cause-and-effect aspects of a social interaction. By reviewing each step of SOCCSS, the child or youth has an opportunity to understand how she makes an impact on the circumstances of which she is a part. The components of SOCCSS include Situation (define the details of the interaction), Options (consider the choices that are available within the given encounter), Consequences (identify an outcome based on each choice made), Choices (pair the option and consequence statements determining which is most appropriate to obtain the desired result for the given encounter), Strategies (develop a plan based on the option/consequence pair), and Simulation (practice the plan before its actual implementation).

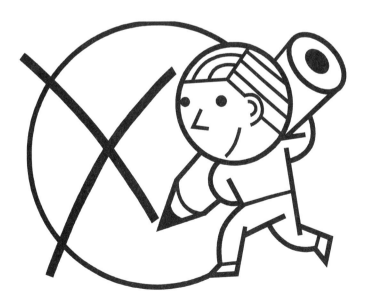

SOCCSS Worksheet
Situation – Options – Consequences – Choices – Strategies – Simulation

Situation	
Who	
What	
When	
Why	

Options	Consequences	Choices

Strategy – Plan of Action

Simulation		Select One
1. Find a quiet place, sit back and imagine how your Situation would work (or not work) based on the various Options and Consequences.		
2. Talk with a peer, staff, or other person about your plan of action.		
3. Write down on paper what may happen in your Situation based on your Options and Consequences.		
4. Practice your Options with one or more people using behavior rehearsal. Start simple and easy for learning. Only make it difficult to test the learning.		
5.		

Simulation Outcomes

Followup

From Myles, B. S., & Adreon, D. (2001). *Asperger syndrome and adolescence: Practical solutions for school success* (pp. 112-113). Shawnee Mission, KS: Autism Asperger Publishing Company. Reprinted with permission.

✓ **Social Autopsy** – Use this strategy to review a social encounter by having the child or youth define what occurred, what went wrong, who was affected, and what could be done differently the next time. Conducting social autopsies is useful because it helps the child identify the social error she made and reiterates that other people are affected by the actions that she takes. It provides the opportunity to problem solve and determine what adjustments ought to be made for future social encounters.

Social Autopsy Worksheet

What happened? _____

_____

_____

What was the social error?	Who was hurt by the social error?

What should be done to correct the error? _____

_____

_____

_____

What could be done next time? _____

_____

_____

_____

_____

From Myles, B. S., & Adreon, D. (2001). *Asperger syndrome and adolescence: Practical solutions for school success* (p. 109). Shawnee Mission, KS: Autism Asperger Publishing Company. Reprinted with permission.

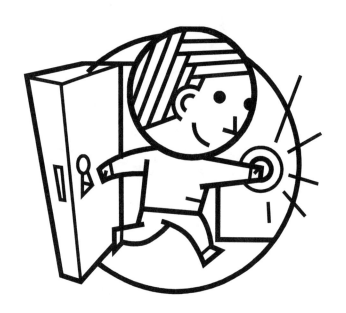

Self-Regulation

When it comes to self-regulation, individuals with AS are challenged on several fronts. First, they experience differences across all the sensory systems (see the following overview of the sensory systems), which may manifest in being either over- or under-sensitive to various stimuli. That is, children and youth with AS may be sensitive to touch, certain types of lighting, temperature, specific sounds, food, holding their head upside down to pick up books, etc. However, they may also lack sensitivity to or awareness of stimuli. For example, students with AS may not know how much pressure to use in holding open a heavy door, when shaking another's hand, in pushing down to write with a pencil, or when lifting a backpack (all proprioceptive – see page 12).

In addition, they often cannot detect that they are upset, anxious, getting too "revved up," and so forth. When asked if they are upset or uncomfortable, therefore, a student with AS may reply in the negative, yet soon thereafter experience a tantrum, rage, or meltdown. To complicate matters, children with AS often do not show the same affect as others when under stress or anxiety. For example, they may show no outward signs that they are getting upset, whereas other kids may complain, yell out, walk away from the situation, and so on.

Failing to interpret their true emotional and sensory state, teachers or other adults may try to teach children and youth with AS necessary skills at times when they are upset, tired, or anxious. This is ineffective because *students with AS cannot learn new skills when stressed or anxious*. An important distinction must be made here: This does not mean that they are not able *to recite* the new skill – only that they cannot *use* the skill.

Sensory Systems: Location and Functions

System	Location	Function
Tactile (touch)	**Skin** – density of cell distribution varies throughout the body. Areas of greatest density include mouth, hands, and genitals.	Provides information about the environment and object qualities (touch, pressure, texture, hard, soft, sharp, dull, heat, cold, pain).
Vestibular (balance)	**Inner ear** – stimulated by head movements and input from other senses, especially visual.	Provides information about where our body is in space, and whether or not we or our surroundings are moving. Tells about speed and direction of movement.
Proprioception (body awareness)	**Muscles and joints** – activated by muscle contractions and movement.	Provides information about where a certain body part is and how it is moving.
Visual (sight)	**Retina of the eye** – stimulated by light.	Provides information about objects and persons. Helps us define boundaries as we move through time and space.
Auditory (hearing)	**Inner ear** – stimulated by air/sound waves.	Provides information about sounds in the environment (loud, soft, high, low, near far).
Gustatory (taste)	**Chemical receptors in the tongue** – closely entwined with the olfactory (smell) system	Provides information about different types of taste (sweet, sour, bitter, salty, spicy).
Olfactory (smell)	Chemical receptors in the nasal structure – closely associated with the gustatory system.	Provides information about different types of smell (musty, acrid, putrid, flowery, pungent).

Finally, individuals with AS do not inherently know what to do to self-calm, refocus, or relax. In the absence of knowing how to return to a typical state of mind, the child with AS is often the victim of tantrums, rage, and meltdowns. The following graphic depicts this escalation of emotion, using the metaphor of a mountain.

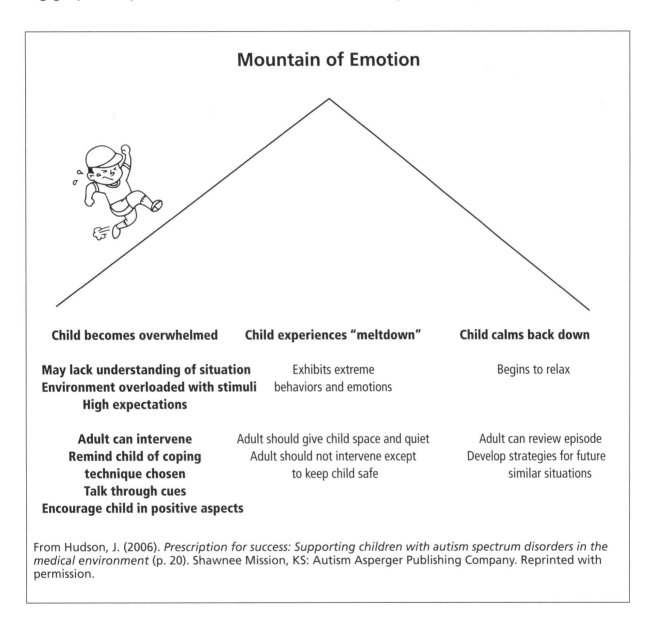

Mountain of Emotion

Child becomes overwhelmed	Child experiences "meltdown"	Child calms back down
May lack understanding of situation **Environment overloaded with stimuli** **High expectations**	Exhibits extreme behaviors and emotions	Begins to relax
Adult can intervene **Remind child of coping technique chosen** **Talk through cues** **Encourage child in positive aspects**	Adult should give child space and quiet Adult should not intervene except to keep child safe	Adult can review episode Develop strategies for future similar situations

From Hudson, J. (2006). *Prescription for success: Supporting children with autism spectrum disorders in the medical environment* (p. 20). Shawnee Mission, KS: Autism Asperger Publishing Company. Reprinted with permission.

Sensory and behavior issues must be addressed as a part of the child's program because research points to these issues as being a continuing part of an individual's life.

Strategies for Self-Regulation

☑ **Sensory Preferences** – Work with parents, others who know the child well, and the child herself to create a list of sensory and related issues that can create discomfort in the child. Ensure that all adults have this list and that the child herself knows the list. In the same manner, create a parallel list of items and environments that the child prefers – those that calm, relax, and soothe her. For example, the seam inside the toe of a sock may irritate the child, whereas a tagless t-shirt may be on the preferred item list. Crowded rooms or loud music may be among the environmental factors that cause offense, whereas dim lights or sitting on the floor are preferred features.

☑ **Direct Teaching** – Teach the student how to recognize when he is uncomfortable or upset. Typically, this can be taught as recognizing a behavior. For example, the student can be taught to recognize that when he starts to get overloaded, he begins to bite his nails. Use visual supports, such as pictures, drawings, or videos, to teach these skills. A signal may be created or established that both the child and the adult can use to remove a child from a potential sensory- and behaviorally unfriendly environment.

Also, it is important to directly teach the child strategies he can use to calm himself down. Use a problem-solving strategy, such as SOCCSS (see page 8), *The Way to A* (2006) by Hunter Manasco, which visually depicts the benefits and consequences of two choices that the child must decide between, or *The Incredible 5-Point Scale* (2003) by Kari Dunn Buron and Mitzi Curtis, which tiers a behavior into five concrete levels (1-5) and thereby visually allows the child to see the range of reactions to each behavior. These tools help the child understand the importance of recognizing sensory issues, stress, and anxiety in herself. An occupational therapist can also be instrumental in identifying and teaching such strategies.

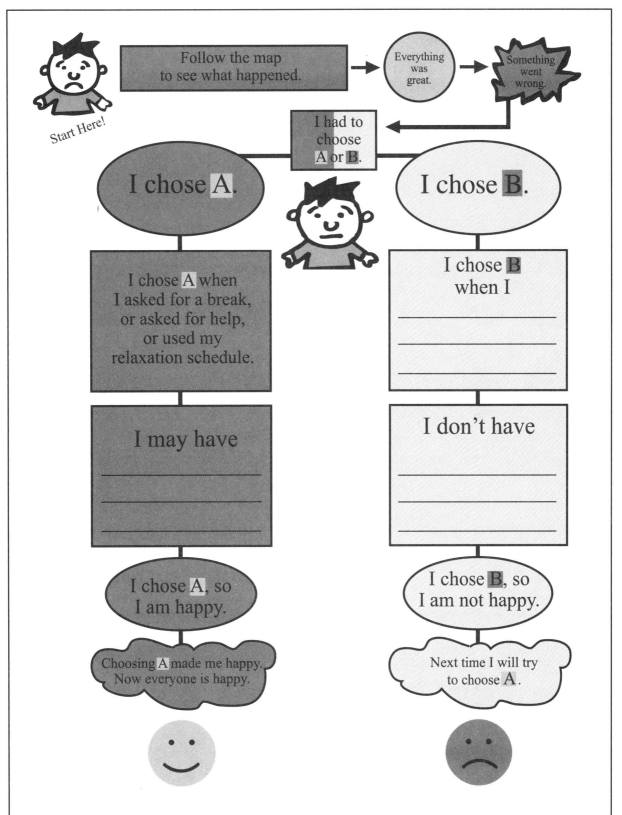

From Manasco, H. (2006). *The way to A – Empowering children with autism spectrum and other neurological disorders to monitor and replace aggression and tantrum behavior* (p. 17). Shawnee Mission, KS: Autism Asperger Publishing Company. Reprinted with permission.

Understanding My Feelings by David

Scared/Afraid

My word for this is:
trembling

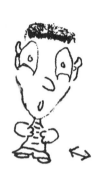

This is how I look:

This is how my body feels:

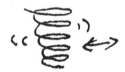

This is what I do:
Hide.

This is what I say:
"I've got to get out of here!"

Things that David says make him "tremble":

"When I get confused."

"When it is loud and crowded."

"Catastrophes like tornadoes and earthquakes and war."

Name: David   My Scared/Afraid/Trembling Scale

Rating	Looks/Sounds like	Feels like	Safe people can help/I can try to
5	Wide-eyed, maybe screaming, and running, hitting.	I am going to explode if I don't do something.	I will need an adult to help me leave. Help!
4	Threaten others or bump them.	People are talking about me. I feel irritated, mad.	Close my mouth and hum. Squeeze my hands. Leave the room for a walk.
3	You can't tell I'm scared. Jaw clenched.	I shiver inside.	Write or draw about it. Close my eyes.
2	I still look normal.	My stomach gets a little queasy.	slow my breathing. Tell somebody safe how I feel.
1	Normal – you can't tell by looking at me.	I don't know, really.	Enjoy it!

From Buron, K. D., & Curtis, M. (2003). *The incredible 5-point scale: Assisting students with autism spectrum disorders in understanding social interactions and controlling their emotional responses* (pp. 42-43). Shawnee Mission, KS: Autism Asperger Publishing Company. Reprinted with permission.

☑ **Home Base** – Provide a home base or cool zone for the child. Create a sensory-friendly environment, taking into consideration all seven senses and where the child can go for a limited time when sensory sensitivity or anxiety occurs. The home base or cool zone is not an escape from school work or other responsibilities. It is relocation to a quiet environment where the child can de-stress and then complete an assignment or any other task.

☑ **Mountain of Emotion** – Teach the student and all adults in the environment to recognize the mountain of emotion and strategies that can be used at each stage (see page 13).

☑ **Self-Calming** – Teach the child or youth a simple relaxation routine such as the following:
1. Take three long breaths.
2. Stretch your arms up over your head, down, and up again.
3. Rub our hands together and count to 3.
4. Rub your thighs and count to 3.
5. Take another long breath.

From Buron, K. D. (2006). *When my worries get too big! A relaxation book for children who live with anxiety.* Shawnee Mission, KS: Autism Asperger Publishing Company. Reprinted with permission.

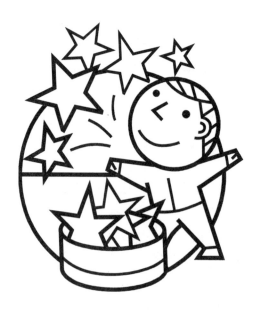

Structure and Predictability

Children with AS enjoy predictability, routine, and sameness. It gives them a sense of logical management and certainty over their day. Therefore, if something is out of the ordinary, whether it is as seemingly simple as an item that is stored in a new place or an event that is added to the daily schedule, it might cause anxiety, confusion, and frustration. That is, when the child is unable to predict what will occur next, the result is a sense of discomfort and worry, which intensifies as the typically predictable circumstance lessens.

A similar reaction to the unexpected may also be observed in interactions with others. Often individuals with AS have narrow special or unique interests as well as a single frame of reference – their own. Both of these characteristics lead the child to believe that his perspective or bank of knowledge is not only correct, but sometimes is the only point of view. So again, if someone challenges his point of view or disagrees with him, it may be difficult for him to be flexible and adapt to the new perspective being presented (refer also to Seeing the Big Picture).

For some of the same reasons, transitioning from one activity to the next is often difficult, especially if there is not much warning or advance notice. Forewarning that an interruption is coming or that the conclusion of an activity is near allows the child to predict the change and to plan in advance for a variation of the schedule. Strategies to prime the individual and assist him in predicting will decrease the degree of uncertainty and, therefore, equip him to function better throughout the day.

Strategies for Providing Structure and Predictability

☑ **Verbal Priming** – Provide detailed information in advance of an activity. Priming can occur as part of a bedtime routine to review the schedule of activities for the next day; it may occur in the morning when the child first arrives at school; or it may occur immediately before a change in the schedule. If the child is accustomed to receiving frequent updates about daily activities, he will be less surprised when the schedule must be altered. In addition to receiving the news about the change, he also receives information about what will occur instead. This allows the child to continue to feel comfortable about the stability of the changing schedule.

☑ **Social Narratives** – Write stories that provide information about an upcoming scenario in which the child with AS will participate. These narratives may be written in the first person – from the perspective of the child – or in third person – from the perspective of a character encountering the same experience. Both types of stories give detail about the social scene, including details of the environment, the hidden curriculum (unwritten social rules), and the choices available in a given situation. For some children, accompanying the text with pictures enhances comprehension due to the visual learning style of many on the autism spectrum.

Example Social Narrative – Birthday Party at the Bowling Alley

I am going to a bowling alley tonight for a birthday party. When I arrive, I may see many children from my school. I will also see Devon, because it is his birthday. While I am at the birthday party, we will eat cake, watch Devon open his presents, and bowl a few games. The bowling alley will probably be loud because of the bowling balls crashing into the pins. If I feel overwhelmed because of the noise, I can tell Devon's mom and then go to the quiet room for a little while. When the party is almost over, my mom will come inside to get me. She will watch me bowl and wait for me to finish so I don't have to leave before the end. I will be sure to tell Devon "Happy Birthday!" and thank him for inviting me to his party.

☑ **Predictability** – Teach the individual how to predict what will come next or what might occur in a given situation. This is an invaluable skill as it will allow her to stay calm, identify choices, and problem solve during a time that otherwise may seem unpredictable and upsetting. There are several ways to practice predictability.

- **Play the "What if ..." game** – This game creates a continuous brainstorm and elaborates on fictional events that could occur in the child's future. For example, What if … it rains … and we cannot go to the playground today? The child determines several responses to the question. Responses may be written down and reviewed, or the game may be played verbally when writing utensils are not available. For continued predictability, take one of the child's responses and continue to brainstorm alternatives. For example, to the response "We could play games in the classroom," ask "What if two people want to play the same game and we only have one?"

- **Use a Countdown** – Provide the child with a series of numbers or a timer that counts down the amount of time that is left for a given activity. When the time runs out or the numbers get to zero, this signals to the child that the conclusion of an activity has arrived and that it is time to move to the next item on the schedule.

5	4	3	2	1

- **Provide a Waiting Plan** – Waiting is difficult for many individuals with AS. Creating a plan, equipped with a rough estimate of the time frame, as well as activities to engage in while waiting, gives concrete information to an otherwise abstract idea of what may appear to be endless stalling between activities. By defining waiting as a part of the schedule, individuals with AS are not only able to predict that it will come, they also have a plan for how to spend the time. During a time of waiting, using a combination of the above strategies will prove helpful. This may include using a visual countdown of the time remaining and a social narrative describing what will occur during and after the waiting period.

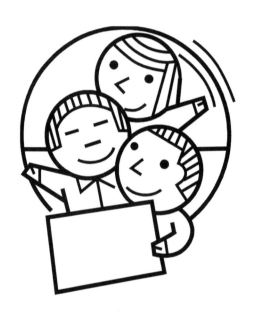

Understanding the Thoughts and Feelings of Others

Detecting Nonverbal and Other Subtle Messages

Social reciprocity – the give-and-take in communicating and interacting with others – is a core deficit among individuals with AS. Being able to identify and interpret the many subtle components of communication is essential for understanding what is being conveyed. Therefore, deficits in this area can seriously impact interactions with others.

For example, recognizing nonverbal cues during a conversation is necessary for fully understanding the verbal words being spoken, as the same phrase may be said with different inflections, facial expressions, or attitudes and, therefore, with completely different meanings. Nonverbal cues such as facial expressions, body posture, and gestures all play a role in communication. They convey the thoughts, feelings, and intentions of others and guide our response to those with whom we interact. Individuals with AS must be taught how to recognize nonverbal cues as well as how and when to respond to them.

In addition to recognizing such cues from others, children with AS must also be taught the messages they send through their own posture, facial expression, proximity, and gaze. Demonstrating how to use the body to express feelings or to show that they are listening will assist children with AS in accurately conveying their intended message.

Lastly, individuals with AS are typically literal interpreters of words and often do not easily recognize idioms, metaphors, slang phrases, or sarcasm. For example, when Manuel greeted John by saying "What's up?," John did not realize that this phrase was common slang for "hello". Puzzled, John thought this was an unusual question, but answered it nonetheless with a literal response, "the sky."

Social interventions must be directly taught to students with AS. Interventions are most effective when embedded into the child's typical routine because that way the child comes to recognize that social interactions are not routine or consistent. They vary and are flexible, depending on the situation. When skills are only practiced by rote memorization or a repetitive method, they are learned, but are not necessarily generalized to situations beyond the setting where they were initially taught. By providing the child opportunities to learn in real-life situations, we enable him to gain experience and skill in his natural routine – in places and with people that he will likely encounter again and again.

 Strategies for Understanding the Thoughts and Feelings of Others

☑ **Direct Teaching** – Introduce nonverbal signs that are familiar to the child, such as waving hello, motioning "come here," or shaking the head to say "no." Identify other less well-known nonverbal cues as they are used in conversations or in magazine pictures and determine with the student what is being conveyed through the gesture or expression.

☑ **Charades** – Have each member of a group take turns acting out predetermined scenarios, exaggerating nonverbal gestures and expressions. Continue acting until a member of the group has accurately guessed what is being conveyed. This activity can also be done silently, using only nonverbal gestures.

☑ **Group Role-Play** – Pick a scenario, such as losing when playing a board game, and discuss various reactions that one might have. Encourage the individual to think how to appropriately respond when each circumstance occurs – interpreting the thoughts, feelings, and reactions of others. Role-play the scene several times, changing the reactions and response to the situation or changing each person's role in the scenario.

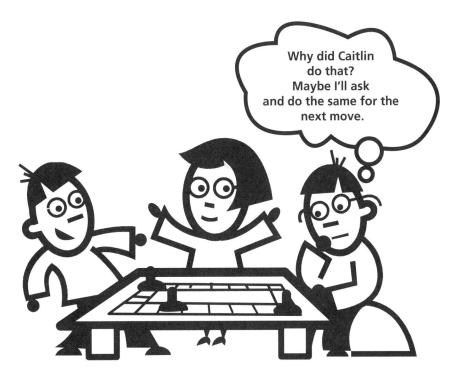

☑ **Comic Strips** – Use blank comic strips as a review of a situation where it was difficult for the child with AS to understand and respond to the nonverbal communications being conveyed. Have her draw one idea in each of several squares depicting the interaction. Discuss what possibly occurred and where the miscommunications took place. Then have her draw a new comic strip as a way to decide what could be done differently the next time. It is not necessary to be good at drawing. Stick figures are fine.

Example Comic Strip Conversation

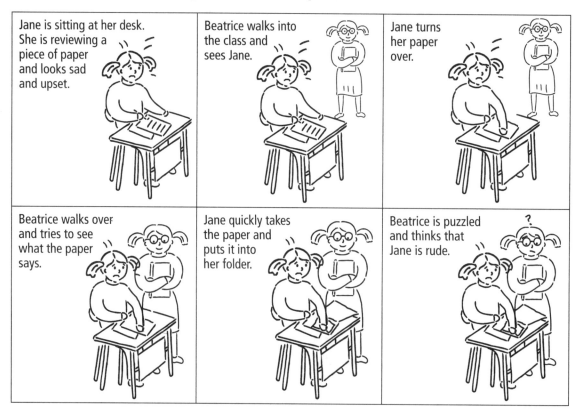

Instead, next time try:

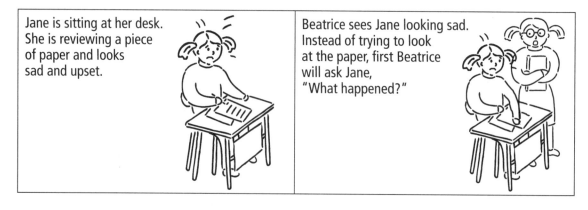

Getting Along
with Others

Social Interactions

Most children and youth with AS want to be a part of conversations and to interact with others, but they struggle with knowing how to join in. Also, once they have joined in, they have difficulty maintaining their part of an interaction. Some abruptly push their way into a group, dominating the conversation with information about their favorite topic. Others may feel over-whelmed at having to decide the right time to join a conversation and, therefore, initiate very awkwardly or not at all. These difficulties often lead to the child being excluded and feeling isolated and alone.

Even the most basic interactions with others involve some form of conversation. Conversations are complex, consisting of multiple aspects, such as beginning a dia-logue, maintaining a mutual give-and-take, listening, following the flow of topics, as well as bringing the interaction to a close and exiting. Understanding and being able appropriately to apply the mechanics of conversation is central to the success-ful participation of individuals with AS.

Individuals with AS typically have narrow, special interests about which they know a great deal of important as well as not-so-important facts. However, these topics may not be the most stimulating or interesting to whomever the child with AS happens to be interacting. Therefore, he may need assistance in determining appropriate topics of conversations and how, when, and for how long to talk about his special interest.

Without being able to understand how to navigate an interaction, an individual with AS may dominate the conversation. Determining ways to segue into a topic or to comment on a current conversation topic are ways to enter a conversation successfully. In the same way, ending a conversation or interaction may be difficult. The child and youth may not recognize the nonverbal cues from others that indicate the conversation is coming to a close. If oblivious to these cues, she may continue to talk, unintentionally prolonging the interaction. Conversely, if an individual with AS decides that he is done with a conversation or interaction, he may simply walk away or stop talking and start on another task, unaware of the need for a closure statement indicating that he is finished. Either way, these behaviors are likely to cause the conversational partner or group to exclude the child with AS instead of embracing him into the interaction.

Social interventions must be directly taught and are more effective when they are embedded into the child's typical routine, as mentioned earlier. By providing the child opportunities to learn in "real-life" situations, we enable him to gain experience and skill in his natural routine – in places and with people that he will likely encounter again and again.

Strategies for Successful Social Interactions

☑ **Scripting** – Write out sentence starters or full scripts to give the individual with AS a visual prompt to use as he engages with others. Creating a list of conversation topics or questions to ask may be helpful as well.

☑ **Turn Taking** – Teach children with AS the basic skill of turn taking as a way of improving her social interactions. The following is a simple and enjoyable way of getting the concept of turn taking across. Toss a ball when engaging the child in casual conversation at home and explain that when she is holding the ball, she can speak. In order to pass the ball to another person, she must first engage in a conversation. Pass the ball back and forth, speaking on variety of topics chosen by all the members of the group. Ask questions, make comments, use names, and flow with various topic changes. Also, as other games (such as board games) are played that call for one person at a time to make a move or take a turn, reiterate the skill of turn taking and responding appropriately.

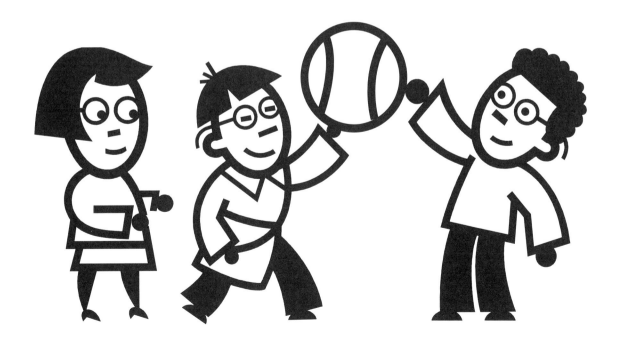

☑ **Direct Teaching** – Break down each component of a conversation or interaction to make them more approachable and easier to understand. Focus on one skill to teach, such as exiting an interaction. Provide reasons why each component is important and role-play several scenarios to practice the skill. More important, embed these skills into the daily routine as the child interacts with those around him.

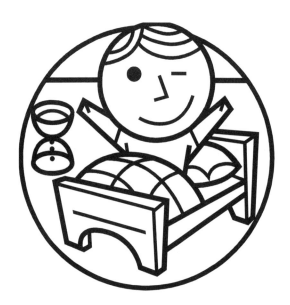

Unwritten Rules

Individuals with AS do well when information is spelled out and presented in detail. However, when faced with knowledge that is assumed to be familiar or is unwritten, they often run into problems. This is referred to as the "hidden curriculum" – the unstated dos and don'ts of everyday behavior that most everyone, except children and youth with AS, seems to know. The hidden curriculum encompasses behaviors, modes of dress, and so on, across situations that most people learn more or less by osmosis and, therefore, take for granted. Every school and every society has its own hidden curriculum. Due to its subtlety and changing nature, this unspoken curriculum causes challenges and, indeed, grief for those with AS.

To illustrate the complex nature of the hidden curriculum, let's use the example of the hidden curriculum for talking to and/or taking rides from strangers. The general rule is: *Never talk to or accept a ride from a stranger*. Unfortunately, it is not that simple. The bus driver is a stranger, but it is permissible to accept a ride from her. It is not okay to ride with the stranger who pulls up to the curb and stops. The cashier at the grocery store is a stranger, but it is acceptable to make small talk with him, but it is not okay to divulge personal information to someone who is standing in the produce section.

The cost of failing to understand the hidden curriculum is sometimes no worse than an awkward moment or a snigger, but other incidents can have more grave consequences. For example, individuals with AS need to learn that they are never to argue with a police officer. They also need to know: (a) teacher expectations,

(b) students to interact with and those to stay away from, and (c) behaviors that attract both positive and negative attention. Other "sensitive" topics of assumed information should be discussed as well, including sexuality, dating, white lies, etc. Understanding the hidden curriculum can make an enormous difference to individuals with AS over a wide range of situations – it can keep them out of detention and can help them make lifelong friends.

Students with AS are at a disadvantage because they do not understand the hidden curriculum. As a result, they inadvertently break unwritten rules and either get in trouble with adults or become ostracized or hurt by peers. To avoid such problems, instruction on hidden curriculum items should be an integral part of the education of children and youth with AS.

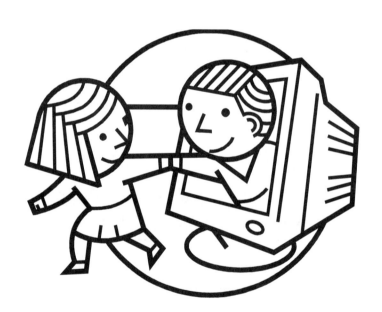

Strategies for Teaching and Integrating the Hidden Curriculum into Everyday Life

 "One-a-Day" Method – Build into the daily schedule a time to discuss one hidden curriculum item from a source such as *The Hidden Curriculum Calendar (www.asperger.net* or Raymer and Scheuer's *Staying Home Alone: A Girl's Guide to Feeling Safe and Having Fun* (these rules also apply to boys). The item may be presented at home during breakfast or the morning routine or at school written on the white board and shared with the class or presented after lunch.

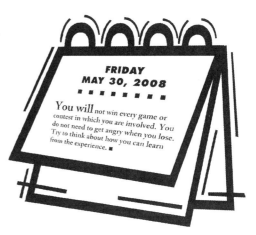

 Teachable Moments – Recognize the appropriate moment to teach a hidden curriculum item. For example, before a field trip that includes standing in line, remind the students about the protocol for standing in line with others. Also, integrate discussions of the hidden curriculum into academic subjects. For example, when reading history texts, identify the unwritten rules that existed at a given time but that may not apply today. Or when studying another country, compare its hidden curriculum to that of the United States (e.g., belching after a meal is considered rude in this country, but in China it means that you appreciated a good meal).

 Child-Friendly Reading Materials – Have children read books that naturally incorporate hidden curriculum items, such as *How Rude! The Teenager's Guide to Good Manners, Proper Behavior, and Not Grossing People Out* by Alex Packer and the *American Girl Series* by the Pleasant Company. Also, direct the child to magazines and periodicals that discuss the hidden curriculum, such as *Real Simple, Reader's Digest, American Girl Magazine*, the Boy Scout handbook, or *Discovery Girls*. These commonly available materials provide information for all children and adolescents in a manner that is simply laid out and easy to navigate.

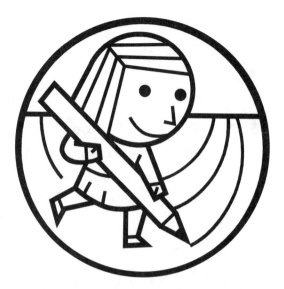

☑ **Hidden Curriculum Journal** – Have students keep a log entitled "One Interesting Fact and Social Skill I Learned Today." Encourage students to share their information. Interview same-age students and ask them what it takes to be successful with peers and adults. Provide this knowledge to students with AS.

☑ **Do-Overs** – Incorporate the concept of Do-Overs into the curriculum. Tell all students, including those with AS, that everyone makes social mistakes and when this occurs, it is important to allow everyone a second chance, a Do-Over. Have the child with AS write about the social error as well as how to correct it or do it differently the next time. (See also social autopsies on page 9.)

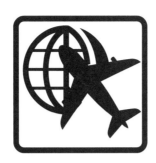

Making a Special or Unique Interest Work for a Child or Youth with AS

One of the criteria for diagnosing AS listed in the *Diagnostic and Statistical Manual of Mental Disorders* (DSM-IV, TR), a guide commonly used in the United States to diagnose Asperger Syndrome, is "restricted and repetitive interests." For children and youth with AS, this often appears as unique or special interests. These interests can be long-lasting or temporary and can include mundane as well as usual topics. For example, we have known children with AS whose interests have included animation, the Flying Tigers, washing machines, the Revolutionary War, the reproductive system, Social Security, videogames, and mass transit systems.

> Emo's special interest was baseball cards, and his collection exceeded 1,500 cards, many of them quite valuable. He carefully catalogued and stored them, and he talked about them incessantly, whether his listeners appeared interested or not.

Often adults try to redirect children and youth with AS from thinking or talking about their special interests because their preoccupation may interfere with interacting with potential friends or distract from completing activities (such as school work). While it may be necessary to curb a near-obsessive special interest at times, it is important to recognize the significance that individuals with AS place on their special interests. In fact, research has shown that people with AS often define themselves by their interests.

> Mia proudly exclaimed to everyone she knew, "I am a junior entomologist! People know I am smart because I know everything about insects." For students like Mia, who are often isolated and feel inadequate, this is a great confidence booster.

Special interests also serve as strong motivators for individuals for whom little else serves as a reinforcer.

> Jeff's teachers had tried every traditional reinforcer they could think of, to no avail. It was not until they turned to his special interest, Pokémon, that they were successful in motivating him to complete less preferred tasks. Jeff did not need to receive a card for each task completed; allowing him time to talk about Pokémon was a powerful reinforcer in itself.
>
> Jem did not like composition even when given a computer for assignments. However, when allowed to write about his special interest, Star Trek, he was able to produce complex essays.

Strategies That Capitalize on Special Interests

☑ **Special Interests and Academic Tasks** – Have the student read books on her special interest, write paragraphs on the topic, conduct Internet and library research, and so forth. Allow the student to use his special interest to learn about topics that might not be of primary interest. For example, the student who is interested in washers and dryers may be asked to investigate how people cared for themselves and their belongings during a unit on the Revolutionary War. The student may also be asked to investigate "mechanical" or similar innovations that occurred during this time period.

☑ **Communicating with Others** – Teach the child how to integrate a special interest into conversations and how to judge how much others want to hear about that topic. For the student who enjoys mass transit systems, for example, it may be appropriate to ask fellow students when was the last time they rode the subway, but then make sure to move on to a topic of more general interest. Also, encourage the child with AS to keep a journal on his special interest and write or draw in it daily.

☑ **Reinforcement** – After a child completes a less preferred task, allow her to spend time at the computer learning about her interest or reading a book on a favorite topic.

☑ **Social Opportunities** – Encourage the child to join clubs or attend outings related to her special interest. The student who is interested in Pokémon can attend Pokémon games and trading sessions often offered at bookstores or community centers. Some universities and junior colleges offer free lectures on various topics. Seek out the pertinent information and encourage the child to attend such special-interest gatherings. Also, focus career days and job internships on the student's special interest.

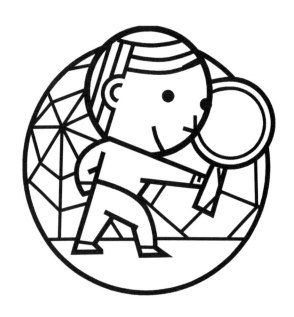

Organization

It is often difficult to understand why individuals with AS have difficulty with organizational skills. Intuitively, it might seem that individuals with AS who are literal thinkers, focus on small details, and like predictability would inherently be organized. However, this is not the case. The root of organizational challenges for children and youth with AS may be found in the definition of organization: *coordinating separate elements into a structure with an implied relationship between separate elements and the coherent whole*. When stated this way, the organizational challenges of individuals with AS become more obvious.

First, as illustrated earlier in this book, a special challenge related to AS lies in understanding *what* the relationship is between details and the whole. In school, the student with AS can list the four types of persecution experienced by early Pilgrims in Europe before they set out for the New World – the details. However, he is not able to link persecution with why the Pilgrims opted for a new lifestyle on a different continent – the whole.

Second, individuals with AS have difficulty understanding *how* details can be integrated to create a whole. In academics, for example, the adolescent may not understand how the North's industrial and the South's agricultural cultures could have led to the Civil War. In organization, the student does not understand *how* designating and using a special place in the locker for a social studies book and a social studies notebook can result in (a) always knowing where materials are, (b) arriving in class on time because there is no need to search all over for materials, and (c) experiencing less stress about finding materials, which can lead to more energy to focus on content subject matter.

Third, as illustrated in earlier sections, students with AS have difficulty understanding assumptions and expectations – *implied* information. For example, in academics, when developing an outline, the term *introduction* implies background information, whereas the term *body* implies substantive content. It is generally assumed that students know these concepts. The sample below provides an example of a student with AS who did not understand this concept.

In organization, students are expected to know what "organize your locker," "clean out your desk," or "put things together" mean. When teachers say, "Look for it," many students with AS who have organizational problems do not know how to strategically go about this task.

Understanding Implied Information in an Outlining Task

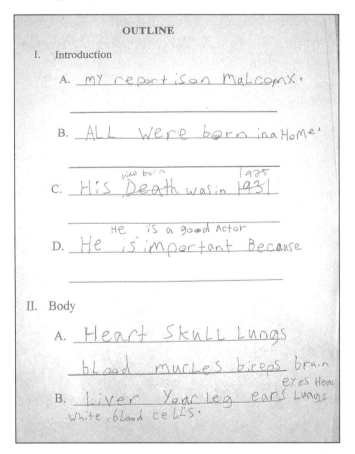

From *Jerri Koeber, Ken Buoy, Kara McHenry, and students, 2007*. Used with permission.

Strategies for Helping with Organization

☑ **Systems** – Think like a professional organizer when working with the child with AS. Establish a system that is easy for him to use, understand, and maintain. This means that everything has one specific place and is carefully labeled. Show the student a picture of what a locker or desk is supposed to look like on the inside, for example.

☑ **Helpful Supplies** – Use color-coding. The math divider in the notebook is red; the math book has a red tab on the spine. Use dividers or folders that have pockets for each subject. Label pockets as work to be completed, work to be turned in, etc. Buy and use locker shelves. Use magazine holders to place in subject matter books and folders. Utilize pencil boxes, pencil pouches, or baggies for small items, such as pencils and highlighters. Make sure that the student who uses a notebook has a three-hold punch in her notebook.

☑ **Routine Support** – Remember that lockers and desks have little to no inherent structure. This means that for students with AS, lockers and desks become vast wastelands where items are misplaced and become difficult or impossible to find. For example, assignments fall to the bottom or are crushed behind books. Schedule times to clean out lockers and desks and teach the student what to keep and what to throw away.

☑ **Classwide Approach** – Spend time the first few weeks of school teaching organization to the *entire* class. Build it into the classroom routine. Also, keep extra pencils, paper, and textbooks in the classroom. No penalty should be given for needing these supplies.

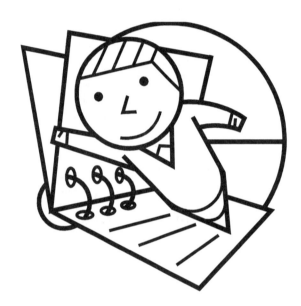

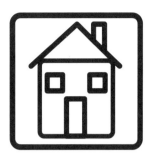

Daily Living Skills

Children with AS often have a delay in adaptive skills and behaviors – those skills needed for successful day-to-day living and adjusting to the world around them. Adaptive skills and behaviors consist of a range of domains and functionalities, including personal skills such as asking a question or requesting help, domestic skills such as tending to a home or caring for personal hygiene, and community skills such as navigating the area to get around independently or participating in a local activity or event.

As mentioned previously, some children with AS have difficulty with taking the perspective of others, which may affect their daily living skills. For example, it may not occur to a child with AS that someone else may have the knowledge or answer to a question he is considering; as a result, he does not seek assistance. Sometimes he may not even recognize a need to ask for help. Without these skills, children may become frustrated, at best, while trying to complete a task single-handedly or finding an answer. At worst, they may give up, consider themselves failures, and lose confidence. In an emergency, failure to ask for help can mean the difference between life and death.

The domestic area of adaptive skills involves self- and home care. Basic hygiene, such as brushing teeth or filing fingernails, can be difficult for individuals with AS due to a sensitive sensory system. Taking a bath or a shower may not seem like a high priority, if it literally causes pain to the skin to wash it. Further, individuals with AS typically have a common disregard for current trends or fashions. They prefer to wear articles of clothing that are comfortable and made of preferred materials that do not irritate their skin. While their comfort should be the number one priority, helping them fit into a peer group by offering suggestions on clothes, etc., is often advisable.

As children get older, adaptive skills include talking on the phone, navigating a map, cooking, cleaning, and caring for a home. These skills are necessary in preparing for independent living. Supports such as visual structuring of the environment by posting signs and labels, breaking tasks into smaller steps, and providing adaptive gadgets and appliances create a user-friendly setting.

It is essential to teach and support the development of adaptive skills and behaviors to foster independence and self-confidence. Due to the core deficits of AS, many individuals do not absorb or refine daily living skills merely by participating in life around them. Further, due to difficulties in generalizing skills and behaviors, it is important to utilize these skills across environments, adapting a skill to accomplish a task.

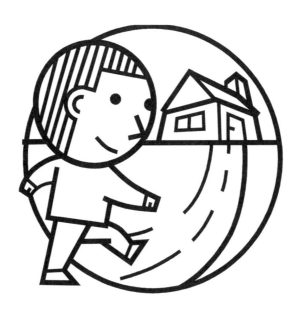

Strategies for Teaching Daily Living Skills

 Breaking Down Tasks – Often a single task consists of multiple steps that must be tackled separately and in a certain order to accomplish the overall task at hand. By breaking down a task into several smaller steps, it seems more attainable and less overwhelming. It also provides information in small increments to ensure that each step is addressed and completed before moving onto the next step.

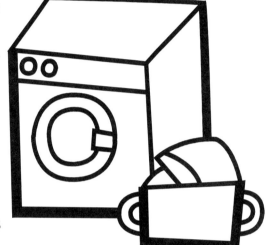

For example, the task of doing a load of laundry seems relatively routine; however, when broken down, it consists of 11 separate steps:

1. Sort the whites from the darks
2. Carry the desired load to the washing machine
3. Select the water temperature and cycle on the washing machine
4. Measure and pour in the correct amount of detergent
5. Load the clothes into the washing machine
6. Start the washing machine
7. Once the clothes have been washed, remember to move them to the dryer
8. Add a dryer sheet
9. Start the dryer
10. Once the clothes are dry, remove from dryer and fold them
11. Put the clothes away

Start by selecting a few steps with which the individual with AS can assist. Gradually, increase the amount of independence and number of steps given to the individual to accomplish. It may take some time before the entire task can be completed independently, but by teaching in small steps, the individual will gain the skills needed to complete the task accurately and be less frustrated.

✔ **Visual Prompts** – Match the child's predominant visual learning style by using visual reminders of the steps/actions that need to be completed. For example, a series of pictures may be taped to the bathroom mirror as follows.

Before going to bed:

1. Brush your teeth	2. Wash your face	3. Take your medicine
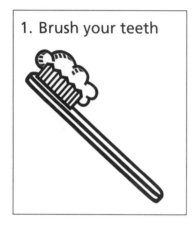	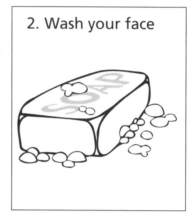	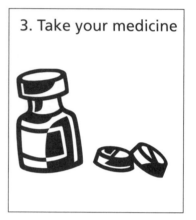

A similar list may be taped by the telephone.

When taking a message:

1. Write down the information	2. Ask for the person's name	3. Ask for the phone number
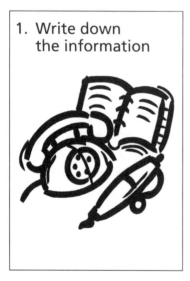	**NAME** 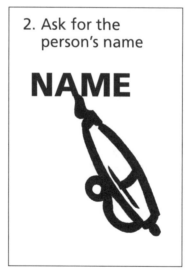	**XXX-XXXX** 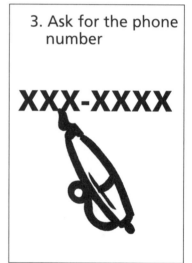

School Subjects

Many academic problems experienced by students with AS are related to the innate characteristics of their AS. Thus, if the teacher is not aware of the student's subtle traits or mannerisms, interventions are often ineffective because they are not addressing the student's underlying needs. The following table outlines some of the characteristics of AS and how they impact learning.

Characteristics of AS and How They Impact School Learning

Characteristic	Example of Impact on Learning
Limited attention span	May miss presentation of content information because thoughts are elsewhere. Because of a lack of awareness that information has been missed, will not seek it out.
Challenges knowing what to focus on and what to ignore	Focuses on how many horses died during Custer's Last Stand and does not understand what led to the event and its outcome.
Problems with reading comprehension masked by average to above-average word-calling skills	When asked a question, can use rote memory to "recite a fact" but has challenges in (a) drawing inferences, (b) sequencing events, (c) understanding cause and effect, (d) interpreting character motivation, and (e) using prediction and other complex reasoning skills.
Motivation to focus on a special interest instead of teacher-directed tasks	When reading about Valley Forge and the American Revolutionary War, focuses on frostbite because it is related to a special interest in weather. Does not understand that his reading goal should be to focus on George Washington's leadership skills during this event.

Characteristics of AS and How They Impact School Learning (cont.)

Lack of understanding of teacher expectations and other unwritten rules	May talk out in class when teacher "expects" the students to be quiet. May not know when the teacher does not want to answer student questions. Does not understand why she cannot be in charge of the cooperative group she is in. When the teacher says, "You cannot ask questions during the examination," student does not understand that she cannot ask content-related questions, but can ask to go up and sharpen pencil.
Poor organizational skills	May miss a math problem because he cannot organize information on the page, such as having difficultly lining up numbers to complete a math operation. Has problems organizing thoughts and creating an outline for a paper.
Difficulty processing auditory information with reliance on visual information to learn	Learns little from teacher oral lectures, particularly when the lecture also contains (a) idioms and metaphors, (b) sarcasm, (c) complex humor, and (d) information that incorporates complex structure and content.
Knowledge of rote (or memorized) tasks instead of conceptual tasks that require an in-depth understanding and manipulation of knowledge	Appears to have a lot of information about a topic but, when analyzed, this knowledge is a recitation of facts and memorized sentences. Often cannot synthesize and apply information. For example, can recite the dates of Shay's Rebellion, its location, and who was involved as well a one or two memorized sentences from the text on this subject. However, cannot understand why this clash threatened to disunite states unless this is directly stated in the text. Also cannot compare and contrast Shay's Rebellion and the Boston Tea Party.
Motor and processing issues that may result in a slower work rate and less production	Focuses on forming letters. Finishes work last with fewer words.
Problems completing homework	Parents may indicate that (a) child needs downtime at home, (b) they do not understand homework, (c) too much time is required for homework, (d) student completes homework but does not turn it in.

Strategies for Implementing Academic Modifications Across the School Day

☑ **Direct Teaching** – Teach content-related information that is helpful across subjects: (a) main idea and supporting details, (b) creating an outline, (c) test-taking skills, (d) using a strategic, detailed charting approach when reading, (e) textbook structure, including where important information is likely to be found (i.e., using a glossary and index, reading chapter summaries, reading captions under figures and tables). A teacher trained in learning disabilities can be helpful here.

☑ **Attention to Important Points** – Accompany oral lectures with graphic organizers that are (a) written on the board or (b) projected on an overhead or projection system and given to the student as a handout. Provide a study guide that tells the student exactly what she is responsible for learning. Highlight information in the text that the student needs to know.

☑ **Task Modification** – Provide teacher lecture notes for the student instead of having her listen and attempt to write notes at the same time. Allow the student to type using a keyboard or other assistive technology device instead of handwriting. Consult with an occupational therapist or assistive technology specialist for assistance. Provide other options than written assignments (i.e., developing timelines, creating a television script, drawings). A teacher of gifted students is an excellent resource here. Use books on tape and/or *Cliff's Notes* to assist with reading tasks.

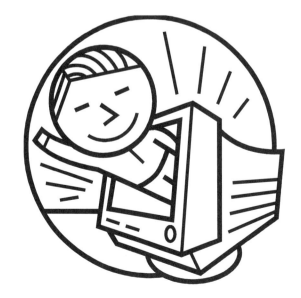

✓ **Structured Tests** – Use a consistent test format; for example, use multiple-choice questions with four options. Allow students to answer test questions orally. If a student provides a wrong answer that appears to be related to a lack of understanding of the content, rephrase the content.

✓ **Models of an Acceptable Assignment** – Work the first problem(s) with the student to ensure that she understands what is to be done. Show a tangible example of a previously completed product or project.

✓ **Specially Designed Work Environment** – Allow students who are easily distracted to complete tasks in a quiet area.

✓ **Homework Modification** – Use your professional judgment when assigning homework. The issue of homework is complex. These and other factors should be considered: (a) how much downtime does the student need at home? (b) how much time should be spent on homework? (c) how will the parents know what homework is required when the student does not have appropriate materials? and (d) what alternative methods can be used to get assignments and materials to families. Reduce the number of problems the student has to do; require only problems that match state standards and that serve as prerequisites for other topics/subjects. The following homework checklist may be helpful. It is important to remember that in some families homework is not feasible – the amount of effort, time, and attention required to start and to then complete the assignments is overwhelming.

Homework Checklist

1. Decide whether to *(check one)*
   - ❑ assign homework
   - ❑ provide a homework time during the day
   - ❑ provide homework based on time to complete, rather than number of problems (time in mins: _____)
   - ❑ eliminate homework (period of time: _____)

2. Select homework planner that has *(check all that apply)*
   - ❑ enough space for the student to write
   - ❑ a specific place to write assignments for each class

3. Decide whether *(check one)*
   - ❑ teacher(s) will provide student with written homework assignment rather than having student write down homework
   - ❑ teacher(s) will prompt the student to write down assignments in planner

4. If the student writes down the assignment *(check all that apply)*
   - ❑ teacher(s) will fill in the missing details student has omitted
   - ❑ specific aspects of homework assignments not written by the student will be identified and a system will be taught for that portion (i.e., due date)
   - ❑ teacher(s) will reinforce student's efforts to write down homework

5. Homework assignments *(check all that apply)*
   - ❑ are presented in written form in the same manner and same place every day
   - ❑ are specific enough so that parents understand the requirements of the assignment solely from the written information provided
   - ❑ include models of assignments whenever possible

6. The home routine for homework completion includes *(check all that apply)*
   - ❑ a designated location free from distractions
   - ❑ a specific time that homework is completed
   - ❑ special considerations for the student (please specify)
   - ❑ use of textbooks that are kept at home for easy reference

7. A method for clarifying homework is in place that includes *(check all that apply)*
   - ❑ a school homework hotline
   - ❑ assignments faxed or emailed to parents at home
   - ❑ a peer buddy who can be called to clarify assignments if needed

8. The plan to monitor completion of and turning in homework includes *(check all that apply)*
   - ❑ having a parent sign the homework planner nightly
   - ❑ parent-assisted organization of homework assignments in backpack
   - ❑ teacher prompt to turn in homework
   - ❑ notify parents weekly of any assignments that have not been turned in

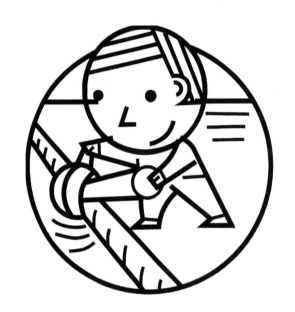

Where to Go from Here

Parents, educators, relatives, friends, and community members are all important people in the life of the child and youth with Asperger Syndrome. The way you create the environment, give encouragement, utilize strategies, and incorporate activities into the child's daily schedule form the basis on which the child learns skills and gains awareness of his own strengths and needs.

While we hope that the descriptions and interventions in this book are helpful to you, they are just the beginning. Therefore, we have provided a comprehensive list of references that provides more detail in many different areas. As you continue to explore the resources available to you, refer back to these pages as a starting point and guide. The information in this book is meant as a simple introduction that we hope provides a foundation as you continue to acquaint yourself with the unique strengths, needs, and characteristics of individuals with Asperger Syndrome.

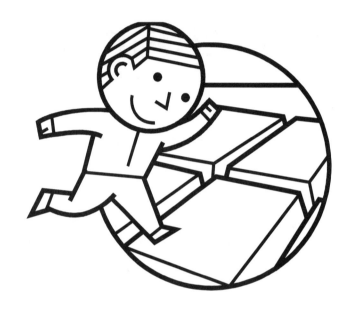

References/Resources

The references underlying many of the strategies and information presented in this book were not incorporated into the narrative to make it easier to read. Instead, they are listed below along with additional resources that we think you will find useful.

Adaptive Behavior

Barnhill, G. P., Hagiwara, T., Myles, B. S., Simpson, R. L., Brick, M. L., & Griswold, D. E. (2000). Parent, teacher, and self-report of problem and adaptive behaviors in children and adolescents with Asperger syndrome. *Diagnostique, 25*(2), 147-167.

Lee, H. J., & Park, H. R. (2007). An integrated literature review on the adaptive behavior of individuals with Asperger Syndrome. *Remedial and Special Education, 28*, 132-139.

Behavior

Buron, K. (2006). *When my worries get too big! A relaxation book for children who live with anxiety.* Shawnee Mission, KS: Autism Asperger Publishing Company.

Buron, K. (2007). *A "5" could make me lose control.* Shawnee Mission, KS: Autism Asperger Publishing Company.

Buron, K., & Curtis, M. (2003). *The incredible 5-point scale: Assisting students with autism spectrum disorders in understanding social interactions and controlling their emotions.* Shawnee Mission, KS: Autism Asperger Publishing Company.

Manasco, H. (2006). *The way to A: Empowering children with autism spectrum and other neurological disorders to monitor and replace aggression and tantrum behavior.* Shawnee, Mission, KS: Autism Asperger Publishing Company.

Myles, B. S., & Southwick, J. (2005). *Asperger Syndrome and difficult moments: Practical solutions for tantrums, rage, and meltdowns* (2nd rev. ed.). Shawnee Mission, KS: Autism Asperger Publishing Company.

Roosa, J. B. (1995). *Men on the move: Competence and cooperation: Conflict resolution and beyond*. Kansas City, MO: Author.

Cognitive and Academic

Arwood, E. L., & Kaulitz, C. (2007). *Learning with a visual brain in an auditory world: Visual language strategies for individuals with autism spectrum disorders*. Shawnee Mission, KS: Autism Asperger Publishing Company.

Hale, S., Pexman, P. M., & Glenwright, M. (2007). Priming the meaning of homographs in typically developing children and children with autism. *Journal of Autism and Developmental Disorders*, *37*, 329-340.

Kana, R. K., Keller, T. A., Cherkassky, V. L., Minshew, N. J., & Just, M. A. (2006). Sentence comprehension in autism: Thinking in pictures with decreased functional connectivity. *Brain*, *129*, 2484-2493.

Killiany, R. J., Moore, T. L., Rehbein, L., & Moss, M. B. (2005). Memory and executive function in autism. In M. Bauman & T. L. Kemper (Eds.), *The neurobiology of autism* (pp. 59-64). Baltimore: Johns Hopkins University Press.

Koshino, H., Carpenter, P. A., Minshew, N. J., Cherkassky, V. L., Keller, T. A., & Just, M. A. (2005). Functional connectivity in fMRI working memory task in high-functioning autism. *Neuroimage*, *24*, 810-821.

Lainhart, J. E., Bigler, E. D., Bocian, M., Coon, H., Dinh, E., Dawson, G., et al. (2006). Do individuals with autism process categories differently? The effect of typicality and development. *Child Development*, *77*, 1717-1729.

Myles, B. S., & Adreon, D. (2001). *Asperger Syndrome and adolescence: Practical solutions for school success*. Shawnee Mission, KS: Autism Asperger Publishing Company.

Steele, S. D., Minshew, N. J., Luna, B., & Sweeney, J. A. (2006). Neuropsychologic functioning children with autism: Further evidence for disordered complex information-processing. *Child Neuropsychology*, *12*, 279-298.

Communication

Klin, A., Saunier, C. A., Sparrow, S. S., Cicchetti, D. V., Volkmar, F. R., & Lord, C. (2007). Social and communication abilities and disabilities in high functioning individuals with autism spectrum disorders: The Vineland and the ADOS. *Journal of Autism and Developmental Disorders*, *37*, 748-759.

Myles, B. S., Huggins, A., Rome-Lake, M., Hagiwara, T., Barnhill, G. P., & Griswold, D. E. (2003). Written language profile of children and youth with Asperger Syndrome. Education and *Training in Developmental Disabilities*, *38*, 362-370.

Sauinier, C. A., & Klin, A. (2007). Brief report: Social and communication abilities and disabilities in higher functioning individuals with autism and Asperger Syndrome. *Journal of Autism and Developmental Disorders*, *37*, 788-793.

Comprehensive Programming

Aspy, R., & Grossman, B. G. (2007). *The Ziggurat model: A framework for designing comprehensive interventions for individuals with high-functioning autism and Asperger Syndrome*. Shawnee Mission, KS: Autism Asperger Publishing Company.

Henry, S. A., & Myles, B. S. (2007). *The comprehensive autism planning systems (CAPS) for individuals with asperger syndrome, autism and related disabilities: Integrating best practices throughout the student's day*. Shawnee Mission, KS: Autism Asperger Publishing Company.

Tsatsanis, K. D., Foley, C., & Donebower, C. (2004). Contemporary outcome research and programming guidelines for Asperger syndrome and high-functioning autism. *Topics in Language Disorders*, *24*, 249-259.

Family Support

Sakai, K. (2005). *Finding our way: Practical solutions for creating a supportive home and community for the Asperger Syndrome family*. Shawnee Mission, KS: Autism Asperger Publishing Company.

General Overview of Asperger Syndrome

American Psychiatric Association. (2000). *Diagnostic and statistical manual of mental disorders* (4th ed., text revision). Washington, DC: Author.

Sensory

Baranek, G. (2002). Efficacy of sensory and motor interventions for children with autism. *Journal of Autism and Developmental Disorders, 32*, 397-422.

Dunn, W., Myles, B. S., & Orr, S. (2002). Sensory processing issues associated with Asperger syndrome: A preliminary investigation. *The American Journal of Occupational Therapy, 56*(1), 97-102.

Green, D., Baird, G., Barnett, A. L., Henderson, L., Huber, J., & Henderson, S. E. (2002). The severity and nature of motor impairment in Asperger's Syndrome: A comparison with specific developmental disorder of motor function. *Journal of Child Psychology and Psychiatry, 43*, 655-668.

Myles, B. S., Hagiwara, T., Dunn, W., Rinner, L., Reese, M., Huggins, A., & Becker, S. (2004). Sensory issues in children with Asperger Syndrome and autism. *Education and Training in Developmental Disabilities, 3*, 283-290.

Myles, B. S., Cook, K., Miller, N. E., Rinner, L., & Robbins, L. A. (2000). *Asperger Syndrome and sensory issues: Practical solutions for making sense of the world.* Shawnee Mission, KS: Autism Asperger Publishing Company.

Pfeiffer, B., Kinnealey, M., Reed, C., & Herzberg, G. (2005). Sensory modulation and affective disorders in children and adolescents with Asperger's disorder. *The American Journal of Occupational Therapy, 59*, 335-345.

Williams, M. W., & Shellenberger, S. (1996). *How does your engine run? A leader's guide to the alert program for self-regulation.* Albuquerque, NM: Therapy Works.

Social

Barnhill, G. P. (2001). Social attribution and depression in adolescents with Asperger syndrome. *Focus on Autism and Other Developmental Disabilities, 16*, 46-53.

Baron-Cohen, S., Golan, O., Wheelwright, S., & Hill, J. J. (2004). *Mind reading: The interactive guide to emotions.* London: Jessica Kingsley.

Bellini, S., & Akullian, J. (2007). A meta-analysis of video modeling interventions for children and adolescents with autism spectrum disorders. *Exceptional Children, 73*, 264-287.

Bellini, S., Peters, J. K., Benner, L., & Hopf, A. (2007). A meta-analysis of school-based social skills interventions for children with autism spectrum disorders. *Remedial and Special Education, 28*, 153-162.

Bieber, J. (1994). *Learning disabilities and social skills with Richard LaVoie: Last one picked ... first one picked on.* Washington, DC: Public Broadcasting Service.

Bock, M. A. (2007). The impact of social-behavioral learning strategy training on the social interaction skills of four students with Asperger Syndrome. *Focus on Autism and Other Developmental Disabilities, 22*, 88-95.

Goddard, L., Howlin, P., Dritschel, B., & Patel, T. (2007). Autobiographical memory and social problem-solving in Asperger Syndrome. *Journal of Autism and Developmental Disorders, 37*, 291-300.

Golan, O., & Baron-Cohen, S. (2006). Systemizing empathy: Teaching adults with Asperger syndrome or high functioning autism to recognize complex emotions using interactive media. *Development and Psychopathology, 18*, 591-617.

Gray, C. (1995). *Social Stories™ unlimited: Social stories and comic strip conversations*. Jenison, MI: Jenison Public Schools.

Gray, C. (2000). *Writing Social Stories™ with Carol Gray*. Arlington, TX: Future Horizons.

Hudson, J. (2006). *Prescription for success: Supporting children with autism spectrum disorders in the medical environment*. Shawnee Mission, KS: Autism Asperger Publishing Company.

LaCava, P. G. (2007). Using assistive technology to teach emotion recognition to students with Asperger Syndrome: A pilot study. *Remedial and Special Education, 28*, 174-181.

Myles, B. S., Trautman, M. L., & Schelvan, R. L. (2004). *The hidden curriculum: Practical solutions for understanding rules in social situations*. Shawnee Mission, KS: Autism Asperger Publishing Company.

Packer, A. J. (1997). *How rude!: The teenager's guide to good manners, proper behavior, and not grossing people out*. Minneapolis, MN: Free Spirit Publishing.

Pleasant Company. (1986-2007). *The American girls series*. Middleton, WI: Author.

Raymer, D., & Scheuer, L. (2002). *Staying home alone: A girl's guide to feeling safe and having fun*. Middleton, WI: Pleasant Company.

Rogers, M. F., & Myles, B. S. (2001). Using social stories and comic strip conversations to interpret social situations for an adolescent with Asperger Syndrome. *Intervention in School and Clinic, 36*, 310-313.

Sansosti, F. J., Powell-Smith. K. A., & Kincaid, D. (2004). A research synthesis of social story interventions for children with autism spectrum disorders. *Focus on Autism and Other Developmental Disabilities, 19*(4), 194-204.

Schultz, R. T. (2005). Developmental deficits in social perception in autism: The role of the amygdala and fusiform face area. *International Journal of Developmental Neuroscience, 23*, 125-141.

Winter-Messiers, M. A., Herr, C. M., Wood, C. E., Brooks, A. P., Gates, M.A.M., Houston, T. L., & Tingsrad, K. I. (2007). How far can Brian ride the Daylight 4449 Express? A strength-based model of Asperger Syndrome based on special interest areas. *Focus on Autism and Other Developmental Disabilities, 22*, 67-79.

APC

Autism Asperger Publishing Co.
P.O. Box 23173
Shawnee Mission, Kansas 66283-0173
www.asperger.net • 913-897-1004